THE HELICOB/
HANDBOOK

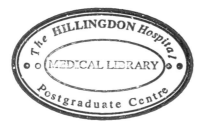

We are overwhelmed as it is,
with an infinite abundance of vaunted medicaments,
and here they add a new one.

Thomas Sydenham MD (1624–1689)

The Helicobacter pylori Handbook

Richard V. Heatley MD, FRCP
Consultant Physician and Gastroenterologist
St James's University Hospital, Leeds, UK

Second Edition

Blackwell
Science

© 1995, 1998 by
Blackwell Science Ltd
Editorial Offices:
Osney Mead, Oxford OX2 0EL
25 John Street, London WC1N 2BL
23 Ainslie Place, Edinburgh EH3 6AJ
350 Main Street, Malden
  MA 02148 5018, USA
54 University Street, Carlton
  Victoria 3053, Australia
10, rue Casimir Delavigne
  75006 Paris, France

Other Editorial Offices:
Blackwell Wissenschafts-Verlag GmbH
Kurfürstendamm 57
10707 Berlin, Germany

Blackwell Science KK
MG Kodenmacho Building
7–10 Kodenmacho Nihombashi
Chuo-ku, Tokyo 104, Japan

The right of the Author to be
identified as the Author of this Work
has been asserted in accordance
with the Copyright, Designs and
Patents Act 1988.

First published 1995
Reprinted 1996 (four times)
Reprinted 1998
Second edition 1998

Set by Excel Typesetters Co., Hong Kong
Printed and bound in Great Britain at
the Alden Press, Oxford and Northampton

The Blackwell Science logo is a
trade mark of Blackwell Science Ltd,
registered at the United Kingdom
Trade Marks Registry

DISTRIBUTORS

Marston Book Services Ltd
PO Box 269
Abingdon, Oxon OX14 4YN
(*Orders*: Tel: 01235 465500
       Fax: 01235 465555)

USA
Blackwell Science, Inc.
Commerce Place
350 Main Street
Malden, MA 02148 5018
(*Orders*: Tel: 800 759 6102
       781 388 8250
Fax: 781 388 8255)

Canada
Login Brothers Book Company
324 Saulteaux Crescent
Winnipeg, Manitoba R3J 3T2
(*Orders*: Tel: 204 837-2987)

Australia
Blackwell Science Pty Ltd
54 University Street
Carlton, Victoria 3053
(*Orders*: Tel: 3 9347 0300
       Fax: 3 9347 5001)

A catalogue record for this title
is available from the British Library

ISBN 0-632-05176-0

Library of Congress
Cataloging-in-publication Data

Heatley, Richard.
  The helicobacter pylori handbook/
    Richard V. Heatley. —
  2nd ed.
       p.   cm.
  Includes bibliographical references
    and index.
  ISBN 0-632-05176-0
  1. Helicobacter pylori infections
    —Handbooks, manuals, etc.
  I. Title.
RC840.H38H43   1998
616.3′3014—dc21   98-24769
                              CIP

For further information on
Blackwell Science, visit our website:
www.blackwell-science.com

Contents

Preface

The last decade has brought many changes to our modern world but few are as great as the impact that *H. pylori* is having on the management of ulcer disease. Not only has this extremely exciting discovery offered new hopes to patients suffering from what otherwise was often a chronic disease, but it has proven extremely confusing to practising doctors faced with claims and counter-claims about the importance of *H. pylori* and what should be done about it.

A variety of review articles and books about *H. pylori* have already appeared but the field is changing so rapidly that it must be extremely difficult for those with their main interest in fields outside gastroenterology to keep abreast of these developments. This must be particularly so in primary care, with so many pressures nowadays apart from simply keeping up to date with all that is new in the different areas of medicine. One of the many problems confounding satisfactory treatment of *H. pylori* infection is continuing confusion over who should be treated and how this is best achieved. I have tried my best to draw reasonably sensible and straightforward conclusions based upon the literature and my own experiences but appreciate that they may not be to everybody's taste!

Having been involved in the production of one of the established comprehensive texts on this subject, and also having contributed to others, I have written this handbook with the generalist in mind. This is intended mainly for those involved in primary care but, hopefully, will also be of value to many in other disciplines including hospital specialities not principally involved with *H. pylori* management, including those in care for the elderly, paediatrics, general bacteriology, chemical pathology, nuclear medicine and pharmacy, as well as others.

I hope that I have succeeded in producing a general text which is of interest to many and in which the information is readily accessible to those who are too busy to read it all but wish to have it as a simple reference source. I am indebted to Pali Hungin and Barrie Rathbone for their helpful advice and constructive criticism.

The success in a very short space of time of the first edition and the rapid developments still occurring in this field have led to this further volume. I am most grateful to all those who have made this possible and to all those who read the first edition and for their many kind comments.

Richard Heatley
Leeds, 1998

1

H. pylori:
the micro-organism

1.1 History links micro-organisms and ulcers

Bacteria have been linked with ulcers for many years

More than a couple of decades ago most people would have shown consternation at the existence of an infective cause for ulcers. This was before the discovery of *H. pylori*, and the subsequent explosion of interest in this area. So much has been written about this in a short period of time that most of us now accept the association, although this was certainly not always the case. Nevertheless, evidence of microbial involvement has been with us for some time: research as long as a century ago linked staphylococci with gastric ulcer development in experimental animals. *Helicobacter* is a spiral organism (Table 1) as are spirochaetes which were first reported in animal stomachs in 1893. During the 1940s human gastric spirochaetes were identified and most appeared to occur in patients with gastric ulcers or cancer. Interest in bacteria as a cause for ulceration then dwindled as reports of viruses in association with peptic ulceration entered the literature. Steer and co-workers renewed interest in bacteria in 1975 but failed to identify the organisms they observed, assuming them to be endoscopic contaminants.

1.2 The discovery of H. pylori

In 1983, three separate groups from around the world more or less synchronously reported the presence of spiral bacteria in patients with chronic gastritis and peptic ulceration. Warren and Marshall from Australia have been ascribed the credit, noting the similarity between these organisms and the genus *Campylobacter*. These curved bacteria were first named *Campylobacter*-like organisms (CLO) but it was not long before they were given the unique term *Campylobacter pyloridis*, later to be changed to

A *Campylobacter*-like organism?

1

Table 1 Characteristics of *H. pylori.*

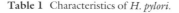

- Major bacterial pathogen found wordwide
- Gram-negative, spiral flagellate
- Microaerophile (requires 5% oxygen), urease producer
- Survives in adverse environments intolerable to other bacteria

Helicobacter is not
Campylobacter

One of several
Helicobacter species

Campylobacter pylori for grammatical correctness. Further work showed biochemical and ultrastructural differences not typical of *Campylobacter* and suggested links perhaps more closely with other species of bacteria, namely *Spirillum* and *Wolinella*. In 1989, the decision was taken by international agreement that this organism in fact represented an entirely new genus, called *Helicobacter*. *Helicobacter pylori*, the 'human' organism, now joins others in the group, including *H. mustelae* from the stomach of ferrets and *H. felis* from cats. These latter are important because they offer hope of animal models for the human disease, where our understanding of the pathogenicity of *Helicobacter* can be investigated and new treatment modalities explored. These organisms are now therefore known *not* to be campylobacters and there is thus *no* link with this common cause of food poisoning.

1.3 The scale of the problem

H. pylori: the
commonest cause
of gastritis!

√ √√

In the relatively short time we have come to know about *H. pylori* a great deal has been discovered about its possible relationship with a variety of gastric and duodenal diseases (Fig. 1). It is now well recognized and accepted that *H. pylori* infection is the commonest cause of gastritis around the world. It is thought to play a major part in the development of peptic ulceration, in particular duodenal ulcer disease. In addition, *H. pylori* has been associated with a number of other conditions in which its role is far less certain. These include gastric cancer and some types of lymphoma, non-ulcer dyspepsia (NUD), lymphocytic gastritis, as well as Ménétrier's disease and protein-losing gastropathy. Some cases of otherwise unexplained chronic abdominal pains in children in the developed countries and childhood diarrhoeal illnesses in the developing world have

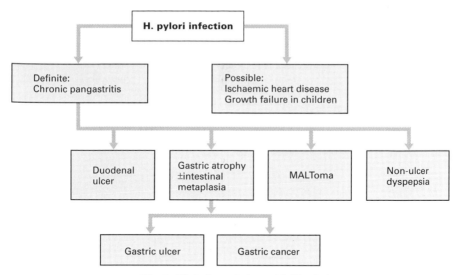

Fig. 1 Clinical associations with *H. pylori*.

also been linked to *H. pylori*. Associations have also been claimed with ischaemic heart disease and reduced growth in childhood in parts of the UK, but these appear very difficult to understand and explain in the light of our current knowledge of *H. pylori*. Since this organism is responsible for one of the commonest infections throughout the world affecting at least half of many populations, it

It affects about half of the population

is perhaps pertinent to examine some of these epidemiological associations critically before reaching firm conclusions about the importance of this infective process.

1.4 Epidemiology

It is a worldwide disease

H. pylori infection occurs throughout the world and it appears that all populations are affected to a greater or lesser extent (Fig. 2). Although detection methods have differed between populations, casting doubt on the validity of some epidemiological findings, a number of important patterns have emerged. However, it must be borne in mind that strain differences may occur between or within individual populations, and serology has often been used in studies based upon antigens of strains taken from completely different countries.

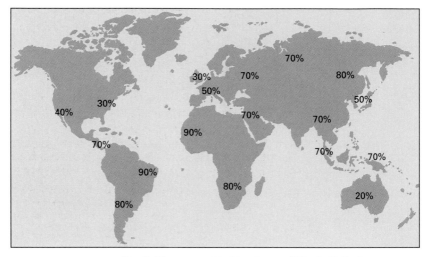

Fig. 2 The geographical incidence of *H. pylori* infection throughout the world.

Infection increases with age

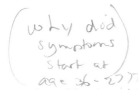

why did symptoms start at age 26–27?

A possible cohort effect

The problem in poorer countries

Infection risks increase with *age*. In all so-called developed countries, the incidence in the indigenous population increases with age, from a low risk in childhood (less than 10%), to approximately half or less of those at 50 years of age. At around the age of 50, the incidence in many studies appears to plateau, perhaps because of the development of gastric atrophy and subsequent intestinal metaplasia within the previously inflamed gastric mucosa, which does not appear to support the continued growth of *H. pylori* (Fig. 3). It is not clear whether this pattern represents a slow and progressive 'spread' of the organism throughout the population with increasing age, or a so-called cohort effect. The latter distribution, an explanation favoured by many at present, suggests widespread infection of the population in the past when living conditions were not so good. This group of infected people have now grown older and the current younger generations are infected much less frequently. This is, of course, only speculation at present, and it will take some time before we are certain of the reason for this distribution.

In developing countries the infection pattern tends to be completely different. In many of the populations studied,

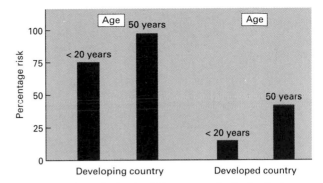

Fig. 3 *H. pylori* infection in different countries (in developing countries most will have acquired the infection by middle age; in the developed world the incidence is much less and may be falling compared with a few years ago).

infection is extremely common in adults, often with up to 90% or even 100% affected. Children in these countries can be infected as early as the first year of life and infection rates as high as 75% at the age of 20 years are not uncommon (see Fig. 3).

Socio-economic factors are probably the other main epidemiological determinant of this infection, apart from age.

Infection commonest in the poor

In general, the poorer populations appear to be at greatest risk. There are also interesting patterns demonstrated within such populations: those that are richer have lower risks of infection compared with the poorest. It has been suggested that childhood crowding is perhaps the single most important risk factor, but undoubtedly availability of clean water and good hygiene standards also have significant effects.

Taking these details into account, there are probably no specific ethnic groups at particular risk, although it has been found in the United States that those with dark skins tend to have the highest infection risks. One interesting group that has attracted attention are Australian Aboriginals.

Aboriginals appear at risk

Those who have had limited contact with white settlers appear to have low levels of infection, but in those who become 'westernized', the rates become extremely high and they also frequently suffer from ulcers.

Groups most likely to become infected

Some studies have suggested that certain groups of workers have higher risks of infection. It has been found that abattoir workers (suggesting an animal source of infection) and even gastroenterologists, endoscoping without using gloves, have high risks. Several different studies have confirmed that infection rates in closed institutions such as orphanages are high, suggesting person-to-person transmission is possible and perhaps especially important in the young.

1.5 Transmission of H. pylori

Where does it live?

The natural reservoir for *H. pylori* is as yet unknown. Apart from living on human gastric mucosa, it is not known to thrive elsewhere. The organism has been found on gastric mucosa in sites other than the stomach. These include: the oesophagus in reflux oesophagitis with a Barrett's mucosa; gastric metaplastic tissue in the duodenum; and ectopic gastric mucosa, for example, in a Meckel's diverticulum and elsewhere in the gut. There have also been claims that the organism can be found in dental plaque in the mouth and in the faeces, but these findings have not been universally confirmed.

H. pylori does appear to survive for a time in gastric juice, and therefore vomiting could be one way that it is spread. In the past, bacterial transmission is known to have occurred during endoscopy with inadequately sterilized instruments. There is also a classic American study where researchers transmitted *H. pylori* infection to a group of human volunteers by means of an intra-gastric pH probe, that was passed from one to another without sterilization.

Passing it around!

Spread in the family

Although it has been speculated that kissing is a means of transmission, there is little evidence for this. Some information points to transmission within families, but this is generally rather sketchy and results are conflicting. At present, it is thought that if transmission does occur in families it may be between adults and children, but is more likely between children. Molecular fingerprinting has been carried out to try and identify intra-familial transmission. Restriction endonuclease DNA analysis has been most used for these purposes. DNA is first extracted from the organism and digested, and the fragments separated on a gel.

Subsequent genetic (chromosomal) patterns can be identified and compared with strains obtained from other infected individuals.

Animals may have it too!

An organism thought at first to be *H. pylori* has been found in domestic cats, non-human primates and pigs. Only the first source is an obvious potential risk for large numbers of the population as a possible reservoir outside the human body, although there are now doubts about this possibility.

Drinking water could be the source in the developing countries

Water is perhaps the most likely medium for transmission in the developing world, particularly if there is any faecal contamination. *H. pylori* has been shown to survive for considerable periods, up to a fortnight, in sea and river water if kept cold. Studies in Peru have concluded that the source of water could be linked very closely with *H. pylori* infection rates. In addition, its epidemiology in parts of the developing countries parallels very closely viruses known to be spread by the faecal–oral route, such as hepatitis A. *H. pylori* has also been found in domestic tap water although it is by no means certain these are viable living organisms.

Swallowing the organism

Human ingestion studies have been carried out involving two individuals who independently swallowed *H. pylori*. The first was carried out by Barry Marshall, one of the first to describe the organism, when he took a suspension of bacteria cultured from a patient, after a dose of acid suppressant. He was previously known to have a normal stomach and an endoscopy 10 days after the organism was taken showed infection and a resultant gastritis. He suffered various non-specific symptoms including borborygmi, epigastric fullness, early-morning hunger, mucus vomiting, headache, irritability and halitosis. By day 14 after infection, 'self-cure' had occurred. A second antipodean, this time a New Zealander, Arthur Morris, carried out a similar study. His account was much more detailed and he developed transient hypochlorhydria. He also had more severe symptoms, mainly colicky, epigastric pain and vomiting. However, he was less fortunate when it came to the outcome, in that it took nearly 3 years and numerous attempts at treatment before eradication of the organism was achieved.

It is interesting to compare this picture with clinical entities outlined by William Osler in his classic medical text-

H. pylori gastritis
has probably been
around for years

book published at the turn of the last century. He described
both acute and chronic gastritis, the latter also being referred to as chronic catarrh of the stomach. The clinical
description bears an uncanny resemblance to what we now
recognize as *H. pylori* gastritis, although, at the time,
dietary indiscretion was thought to be one of the most
likely causes.

1.6 The host response to infection

In addition to the above-mentioned human ingestion
studies there have been individual reports of apparently
spontaneous infections with *H. pylori*. In these, a compos-
ite picture can be formed of the initial acute inflammatory
changes, consisting largely of polymorphonuclear cells,
changing over a matter of months or years to chronic
inflammatory changes with many more lymphocytes.
In parallel, serological evidence of a systemic antibody
response can be observed with, as one might expect, an
early immunoglobulin M (IgM) rise followed much later
by IgA and IgG responses which may slowly fall after eradication of the organism (Fig. 4).

**The inflammatory
response**

The environment in which *H. pylori* colonizes the
stomach is unique in that other infectious agents do not
appear to compete (Table 2). The organism tends to lie
deep in the gastric pits and on the surface of epithelial cells
mainly beneath the protective mucus layer which overlies
the gastric mucosa. It is thought that this location is maintained at a neutral pH, oxygen concentrations are probably
low and essential nutrients are presumably available to the
micro-organism.

Where it lives

There are undoubtedly certain features about the bacterium that make it a potential pathogen. It has been
observed to form microscopic 'adherence' or 'adhesion'
pedestals between itself and the epithelial cell surface,

Table 2 Colonization of the stomach by *H. pylori*.

- Colonizes only gastric epithelial cells
- Gastric antrum is predominant site of colonization
- Uses adhesion pedestals to adhere to gastric epithelium

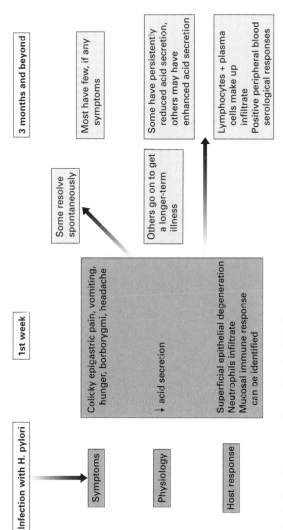

Fig. 4 Probable course of acute *H. pylori* infection.

H. pylori as a pathogen

similar to those observed with enteropathic *Escherichia coli* in the intestine. *H. pylori* also produces enzymes that may be important in causing local cell damage with their proteolytic, and possibly mucolytic, functions. Perhaps the most significant is urease, which converts urea to ammonia, and this may consequently bring about pH changes in the vicinity of the gastric mucosal cells. The organism has also been shown to induce vacuolation (*vacA* gene) or cell death (cytotoxin-associated gene—*cagA*), presumably by production of a toxin, against *in vitro* cell lines. Some strains of the organism have identifiable properties that imply they are particularly pathogenic, such as the *cagA* gene product (a 128-kDa surface protein) reported to be associated with specific clinical conditions, including peptic ulceration. This may explain why not all *H. pylori*-infected individuals develop ulcer disease, although the verification of this theory is complicated by the fact that some patients appear to be infected with more than one strain of bacteria at any one time (Fig. 5). This is further complicated since the proportion of *cagA*-positive strains appear to vary around the world, being particularly prevalent in the Far East.

The body's response to infection

The host responds to these various insults from *H. pylori* invasion by a number of standard immunological defences. Local antibody is produced, cell activation occurs with

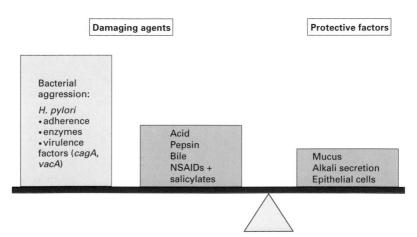

Fig. 5 Balance between potential damaging agents and protection of stomach.

release of soluble mediators (cytokines and chemokines) and subsequent cell recruitment occurs, initially polymorphs, later lymphocytes. Surprisingly, this does not apparently bring about expulsion or death of the organism in all infected individuals. Some organisms deep in the gastric pits appear to evade antibody coating and it is possible this is how the immune response is overcome in some people. Whilst a number of pro-inflammatory cytokines, in particular interleukin (IL)-1, IL-2, IL-6, IL-8 and tumour necrosis factor α (TNF-α) are probably responsible for the recruitment of many different inflammatory cell types, this response does not appear adequate to expel the organism. Simultaneous release of the cytokine IL-10, thought to have a counter-immunoregulatory role, may explain why infection persists in many. This does, of course, raise some questions over the potential for vaccination against the organism in the future, although in animal models, such as *H. felis* infection of the mouse, attempts at immunization have been successful. Vaccination with *H. felis* and adjuvant cholera toxin to enhance the immune response has been shown to protect against later *H. felis* infection of the stomach, which usually causes gastritis in the mouse.

Immunization is possible in animals

H. pylori:
the clinical problem

2.1 Classification of gastritis

Our acceptance now that *H. pylori* is a major causal factor in gastric inflammatory states has revolutionized the way we classify gastritis. Previously, it was understood that autoimmune factors were important in some cases (so-called type *A* gastritis, associated with pernicious anaemia); in others, the causal factor was chemical, including bile reflux and possibly non-steroidal anti-inflammatory drug (NSAID) ingestion (type *C*, 'chemical' or reflux gastritis). Bacteria conveniently fitted into a middle category (*B*-type, '*b*acterial' gastritis) (Table 3). However, it was soon recognized this did not completely encompass all variants and a new classification was borne—the Sydney system. This was more descriptive and included both microscopic and endoscopic appearances in the various categories.

The commonest form of chronic gastritis worldwide is that caused by *H. pylori*. Most of those affected have active, chronic gastritis, meaning that neutrophil polymorphonuclear cells invade intra-epithelial and interstitial compartments, and are accompanied by lymphocytes and plasma cells. Biopsies showing activity (i.e. polymorphs in reasonable numbers) are invariably *H. pylori* positive. *H. pylori* gastritis tends to occur most severely and frequently in the antrum of the stomach, but the body of the stomach can be involved in severe cases (Fig. 6). Other causes of gastritis, namely those due to autoimmunity or a chemical reflux gastritis, are most likely to be *H. pylori* negative. There is one unusual variety of chronic (lymphocytic) gastritis in which the inflammatory infiltrate comprises very much the cell types its name suggests. This is also usually *H. pylori* negative, but there is not infrequently serological evidence of past *H. pylori* infection.

It is now generally accepted that whatever causes the initial damage to gastric mucosa, in the long term, gastritis

Types of gastritis

Pathological changes

Table 3 Autoimmune gastritis vs. *H. pylori* gastritis.

	Autoimmune	*H. pylori*
Morphology		
Gastritis	Corpus	Mainly antral
Gastric atrophy	Eventually	Sometimes
Physiology		
Acid secretion	↓	↓Early, and when atrophy starts
Vitamin B$_{12}$ absorption	↓	No effect
Immune associations		
Associated immune diseases	+	None known
Genetic predisposition	+	None known
Systemic antibodies	PCA	IgM (early acute infection)
	IFA	IgG, IgA (chronic disease)

IFA, intrinsic factor antibody; PCA, parietal cell antibody.

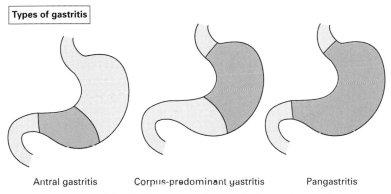

Types of gastritis

Antral gastritis   Corpus-predominant gastritis   Pangastritis

Fig. 6 Changes are often patchy but, at the atrophy stage, this tends to separate into more distinct types. Autoimmune gastritis mainly affects the corpus (body of the stomach), *H. pylori* gives an antral gastritis but, in severe cases, the whole of the stomach may be affected (pangastritis).

may be followed by gastric atrophy, which, in many, can be accompanied by the development of intestinal metaplasia. This is thought by some to be the pathway that could lead to the subsequent development of gastric cancer. Recently, it has been shown that patients with reflux oesophagitis treated with long-term omeprazole who are also *H. pylori* infected appear to develop accelerated gastric atrophy. This is a worry since it may increase the tendency for gastric cancer to develop in these patients, but not all studies have confirmed this finding. Unfortunately, it will probably be many years before this matter is satisfactorily resolved.

2.2 H. pylori, gastritis and non-ulcer dyspepsia

In early *H. pylori* gastritis, the first changes appear to be a neutrophil polymorph infiltrate of the mucosa and these cells may also exude from the epithelial cell surfaces. In chronic gastritis, the cellular infiltrate alters to one predominantly of lymphocytes and plasma cells. Focal collections of lymphocytes as lymphoid follicles is also typical, especially during infection in children and can, on occasion, be identified endoscopically. Glandular loss and atrophy eventually ensue. As subsequent intestinal metaplasia develops, paradoxically *H. pylori* is unable to survive and these individuals may well be negative for the organism when examined. In parallel, the inflammatory response usually settles so that the gastritis no longer appears 'active'.

Long-term changes

Many patients with chronic gastritis often have associated duodenitis and a proportion will suffer dyspeptic symptoms. Since *H. pylori* is frequently associated with these pathological conditions, hardly surprisingly the question has been asked whether *H. pylori* and non-ulcer dyspepsia (NUD) are linked (Table 4). There has often been confusion as to whether gastritis or duodenitis causes symptoms and controversy abounds. A number of studies have shown higher incidences of *H. pylori* infection in patients with NUD than in age- and sex-matched controls. However, many of the results from these studies have been questioned because of difficulties in obtaining adequate data from controls, since dyspeptic symptoms are so common (Fig. 7).

Links with dyspepsia

None of these studies has identified any specific complex of symptoms typical of *H. pylori*-related disease, and the types of complaints patients appear to develop with these disorders vary greatly. There has been speculation that *H. pylori* infection could produce symptoms by affecting gastric acid secretion or upper gut motility, but evidence

Does *H. pylori* cause dyspeptic symptoms?

Table 4 Association of *H. pylori* with non-ulcer dyspepsia.

- *H. pylori* infection is up to twice as common in non-ulcer dyspepsia patients
- *H. pylori* and symptoms: certainly in acute infection, less clear in chronic disease
- *H. pylori* has inconsistent effects on acid secretion and motility
- No definite evidence that *H. pylori* treatment or eradication reduces dyspeptic symptoms

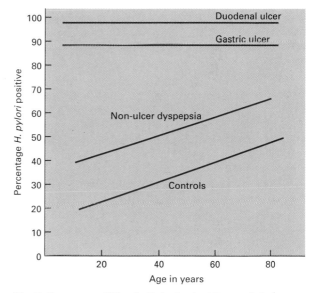

Fig. 7 Frequency of *H. pylori* infection in different clinical situations at different ages.

for both is conflicting. A number of treatment trials have attempted to examine whether *H. pylori* eradication leads to improvement in NUD symptoms. Although, as one might expect, results have not been clear-cut, some patterns have emerged. If *H. pylori* eradication has been achieved satisfactorily, then inflammation in the form of gastritis tends to improve and signs of active inflammation settle. In the short term, a number of studies have shown improvement in dyspeptic symptoms, but large numbers of patients have not been shown to improve in long-term

Treating NUD

H. pylori causes the majority of cases of chronic active gastritis worldwide

- Eradication of H. pylori leads to improvement of the gastritis
- In relation to symptoms and non-ulcer dyspepsia, the role of H. pylori is much less clear

Fig. 8 *H. pylori* and gastritis.

follow-up. A number of the treatment regimens used, particularly those containing bismuth, have mucosal healing properties independent of any anti-*Helicobacter* effects. It may be this mucosal healing rather than an influence on *H. pylori* that leads to an improved symptomatic response (Fig. 8).

2.3 H. pylori and peptic ulcer disease

2.3.1 Duodenal ulceration

The old adage 'no acid, no ulcer' appears to be as true today as previously, but no one can truthfully claim 'no *H. pylori*, no ulcer', since overall, probably 15% of peptic ulcers do not apparently have *H. pylori* infection.

Many patients with duodenal ulceration (DU) have an associated inflammation of the stomach and also the duodenal mucosa—duodenitis. Chronic gastritis, particularly of the antrum of the stomach, has long been associated with DU and it therefore comes as little surprise that interest has focused on the possible role of *H. pylori* in DU disease.

It is now widely accepted throughout the world that virtually all those with DU in the main adult age-range (adolescent through to senility) have *H. pylori* infection of the gastric mucosa. There may be a lower incidence in those from the 'age extremes'. In the few other *H. pylori*-negative ulcers (often about 5%), there is usually some other cause, such as NSAID ingestion or, much more rarely, the Zollinger–Ellison syndrome.

At first sight, it is difficult to understand how an organism that only appears to live on gastric mucosa could cause damage in the duodenum rather than the stomach.

Most DUs are *H. pylori* positive

H. pylori in the duodenum

However, gastric metaplasia has long been known to develop in the duodenum in response to a low pH, usually due to increased gastric acid secretion. This appears to be the route by which those with gastric mucosal infection can be subject to duodenal colonization, the development of inflammation (duodenitis) and presumably later DU (Fig. 9).

The role of H. pylori in DU

H. pylori infection of the stomach is a well-known cause of elevation of serum gastrin which, somewhat surprisingly, does not produce the swingeing changes of increased gastric acid secretion one might anticipate. Subtle changes have been reported in those with DU disease, but the importance of this observation is, at present, unclear.

Apart from host factors leading to possible DU disease, 'virulence' factors related to the organism have been investigated. The feature which has perhaps attracted most attention is the so-called cagA protein, only present with some strains. Controversy surrounds its true role, since some have associated it with gastric cancer, the development of which has long been reported to be less likely in DU sufferers. Variation in the incidence of this apparent marker of pathogenicity around the world may help to explain these apparently contrary findings (Table 5).

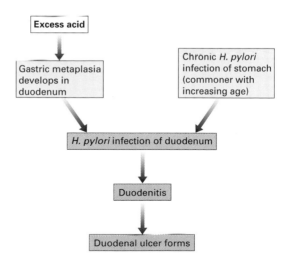

Fig. 9 Likely role of *H. pylori* in duodenal ulceration.

Table 5 Why do only some *H. pylori* patients develop duodenal ulcers?

Host factor?
- Gastric metaplasia in duodenum
- Effects on acid secretion (high parietal cell mass)
- Reduced acid inhibition/atrophy of gastric corpus mucosa

H. pylori virulence?
- Toxigenic strains (*cagA* or *vacA* gene)
- Cytokine release

2.3.2 Gastric ulceration

Gastric ulcers too!

Similar associations have been claimed between gastric ulceration (GU) and *H. pylori*, although most accept that a lower proportion of GU patients have *H. pylori* infection compared with those with DU disease. Gastric ulcers (those found proximal to the antral region) usually tend to develop on a background of pangastritis, with atrophy and intestinal metaplasia frequently found. Apart from *H. pylori*, NSAID consumption is obviously very important in some GU patients. Probably about 75–85% of GU patients can be demonstrated to have current *H. pylori* infection.

After surgery

In ulcer patients who have undergone surgery, *H. pylori* is found in decreasing numbers the more extensive the surgery that has been carried out. Those undergoing vagotomy having the higher levels, gastrectomy the lower. It has been speculated that bile reflux suppresses *H. pylori* colonization of the remaining gastric mucosa.

2.3.3 Evidence linking H. pylori with peptic ulceration

DU after *H. pylori* eradication

The most convincing evidence of a role for *H. pylori* in peptic ulceration is the response of ulcer disease to eradication of the organism. For years it has been recognized that although acid-suppressant treatment rapidly and effectively heals ulcer disease, on discontinuing treatment relapse frequently occurs. A number of studies have confirmed that after successful healing of DU, about 80% recur over 12 months' follow-up and probably 100% relapse over a 2-year period. In the long term, H_2 receptor antagonist treatment reduces the 1-year relapses to about 20–30%. It is now clear that similar success can be achieved without the need to continue long-term treatment by eradicating *H. pylori*. A number of good studies from around the world have shown that after *H. pylori* eradication has been successfully

Long-term recurrences dramatically reduced

achieved, recurrence rates for DU disease over 12–18 months of follow-up are reduced to 20–30%, and some have shown rates as low as 0%. Furthermore, it has been suggested that recurrence over several years' follow-up remains extremely low. It does not appear to matter which original form of treatment was used as long as *H. pylori* is effectively eradicated (Fig. 10).

A similar pattern has emerged for GU patients also, but data are currently more limited in this area and NSAID ingestion probably also plays a major part in causing many GUs (Fig. 11).

One of the major risks of long-standing DU disease is the

Ulcer complications

occurrence of haemorrhage and perforation. Risks of bleeding can be as high as 20% at 15–20 years after an ulcer first presents. Long-term acid suppression in the form of H_2 receptor antagonists has been clearly shown to reduce these risks. There is some evidence to suggest, in the short term, that *H. pylori* eradication treatment may achieve similar effects. Data, however, remain limited and it would probably be unwise to depend on *H. pylori* eradication alone at present to lower the long-term risks of DU disease,

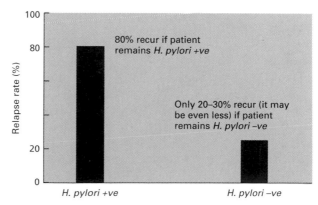

Fig. 10 Relapse rate for duodenal ulcer disease in the first 12 months after treatment.

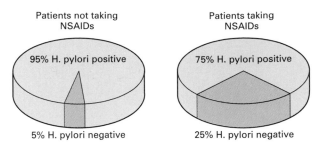

Fig. 11 The effects of *H. pylori* and NSAIDs in patients with peptic ulcer.

a management approach borne out by the National Institutes of Health (NIH) consensus statement. Ulcer perforation does not appear specifically related to *H. pylori* infection and it may be that NSAID ingestion is most important in causing this complication.

Oesophagitis too!

Patients with ulcers do not always remain free of symptoms after *H. pylori* eradication treatment. It is becoming increasingly recognized that they may return with symptoms of gastro-oesophageal reflux disease (GORD)—primarily heartburn. Although *H. pylori* infection appears if anything less frequent in GORD, patients with previous peptic ulceration do appear particularly susceptible to developing symptoms.

2.4 H. pylori and gastric cancer

The gastritis–cancer sequence

There has been an appreciation for some time that chronic gastritis can be a precursor for the development of the 'intestinal' type of gastric cancer. The suggested sequence of events is that gastritis over the years leads to gastric atrophy and intestinal metaplasia. In some individuals adenocarcinoma subsequently develops over a 15–20 year timespan. The acceptance of a form of gastritis linked to *H. pylori* has ranked this form of gastritis along with autoimmune gastritis as pre-malignant conditions (Fig. 12).

Infection rates and cancer risks

However, the relationship between *H. pylori* and gastric cancer is somewhat difficult to prove, since *H. pylori* infection is often difficult to demonstrate in actual stomach cancer specimens because of the presence of gastric atrophy and intestinal metaplasia, which does not support contin-

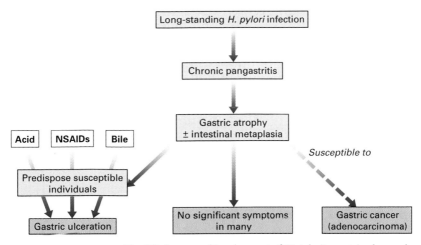

Fig. 12 Suggested involvement of *H. pylori* in gastric ulcer and gastric cancer.

ued growth of the organism. Serological studies have suggested evidence of previous infection in a high proportion of gastric cancer patients. It is, nevertheless, important to recognize that both *H. pylori* infection rates and those of gastric cancer tend to rise with increasing age and lower socio-economic status, and links may be no more than coincidental. In reality, *H. pylori* is probably simply a risk factor for the development of certain types of gastric cancer. It has been estimated from epidemiological studies that this infection may increase the risk of developing gastric adenocarcinoma by 3–6-fold. In some studies, links have been found between high *H. pylori* infection rates and high gastric cancer incidence. Not all have, however, confirmed an association, although in China, for instance, the suggestion has arisen that acquisition of infection at a young age may be what is most relevant. Correlations have been found between serological titres for *H. pylori* and gastric cancer rates in both the Far East and centres throughout Europe and the United States. In the UK, associations between gastric cancer and childhood overcrowding have led to a belief that *H. pylori* infection in children may be significant in later gastric cancer development (Fig. 13).

Not all studies agree there are links

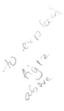

Review article.

21

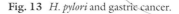

H. pylori appears to possibly play a role in the development of gastric cancer, probably by first causing chronic gastritis

• If this proves to be the case, then widespread eradication programmes will need to be developed

Fig. 13 *H. pylori* and gastric cancer.

Could *H. pylori* be a carcinogen?

In the steps thought to be important in the development of gastric cancer, as glandular atrophy develops and gastric acid output diminishes, bacterial overgrowth may occur. Some bacteria are capable of reducing dietary nitrate to nitrite, which can then form a number of highly reactive chemical species, themselves reacting with dietary amines to form potentially carcinogenic *N*-nitroso-compounds. This whole process can be inhibited by antioxidants such as ascorbic acid (vitamin C) (Fig. 14). Interestingly, large amounts of ascorbate normally appear in gastric juice, but these levels are reduced in *H. pylori* gastritis and what is present is largely inactive. Therefore, an attractive hypothesis forms that *N*-nitrosocompounds may be abundant in *H. pylori* infection and this is what leads to cancer formation. Unfortunately, this turns out not to be proven in the light of current evidence. Other theories have abounded, including the presence of reactive oxygen species, ammonia, cytotoxin-producing strains of *H. pylori* and the presence of cytokines, all of which may be important in inducing carcinogenesis, but few have convincing supporting evidence. Notwithstanding, the World Health Organization has classed *H. pylori* as a definite carcinogen, which has caused great surprise to a number working in the field!

WHO has classed it as a carcinogen

Low-grade B-cell lymphomas

H. pylori has also been linked with other gastric neoplasms, namely the uncommon tumours of gut lymphoid tissues known as mucosa-associated lymphoid tissue (MALT). These lymphomas, or MALTomas, are generally low grade and have been shown to be associated with *H. pylori* infection. Furthermore, eradication of infection has been claimed in a small number of cases to have resulted in tumour regression. Obviously the outcome of long-term follow-up studies involving larger numbers of patients will be keenly awaited.

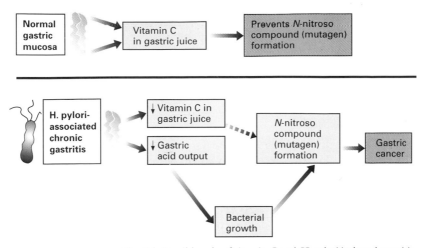

Fig. 14 Possible role of vitamin C and *H. pylori*-induced gastritis in gastric cancer.

Not all bad news!

Despite the association of *H. pylori* with gastric cancer the same may not necessarily be true in the oesophagus. Recent evidence points to a negative association between *H. pylori* infection of the stomach and cancer of the oesophageal cardia suggesting perhaps in this case a protective effect of *H. pylori*.

2.5 H. pylori in children

Affects those with bellyache

Although paediatric infection is common in developing countries, in Europe and North America the incidence is low in most indigenous population groups (<10% of under-16-year-olds). Some have found a higher incidence in those with recurrent abdominal pain, a syndrome thought previously to have important psychosocial features. Those affected often appear to suffer colicky, periumbilical or epigastric pain and sometimes vomiting. About 20–30% of those with otherwise unexplained chronic abdominal pain have evidence of *H. pylori* infection and most had been found to occur in the 8–16-year-old age-ranges in some studies.

Children get it too!

Ulcers can also affect children, albeit less frequently than in adults, and these are often *H. pylori* positive. *H. pylori* has, in addition, been associated with a protein-losing gastropathy in a small number of children. If *H. pylori* infection is diagnosed by serology in childhood, it is important to recognize that titres may be different to those accepted in adults. At endoscopy in children, *H. pylori* infection has been reported to cause antral nodularity, probably because of the development of lymphoid follicles within the gastric mucosa.

Infected children were initially treated with bismuth–antibiotic combinations, mainly amoxycillin or ampicillin and tinidazole. There are, theoretically, grounds for concern over the safety of bismuth since, in the past, a form of encephalopathy has been reported in France, but this has not caused obvious problems in short-term treatment. Data with other combinations are much more limited, and a number of treatments used in adults, such as proton-pump inhibitors, do not have licensed indications for childhood usage but are being used increasingly by those with expertise in this area.

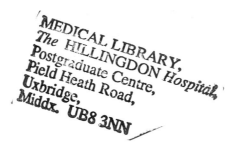

3   Management of H. pylori infection

3.1 Detection of H. pylori

There are a number of both *direct* and *indirect* ways of identifying *H. pylori*. Direct methods involve invasive tests and essentially this means an endoscopy (Table 6).

3.1.1 Direct tests

Endoscopy

Endoscopic appearances of *H. pylori* infection

There are no specific features of *H. pylori* infection seen endoscopically. Inevitably, those with gastritis may have diffuse reddening of the mucosa, but correlation between histology and endoscopic appearances in gastritis are not generally good. Although probably better in the duodenum, once again endoscopic appearances are by no means diagnostic. In children it has been reported that antral nodularity is a feature of *H. pylori* infection, but it is not known how specific these findings are. Diagnostic confirmation of *H. pylori* endoscopically depends upon gastric and/or duodenal biopsy.

Histology

Histology is a reliable method for detection of *H. pylori* infection. The bacteria are spiral and appear curved or S-shaped and are usually plentiful in number, particularly in the antrum of the stomach where they are frequently most numerous. They most commonly lie close to the surface of epithelial cells and are often present in the overlying gastric mucus.

Staining characteristics

When first identified, special stains were needed and originally the Warthin–Starry silver stain was used by many. However, most practised histopathologists will now recognize the bacteria using Giemsa stain and can often even

Table 6(a) *H. pylori* tests.

Invasive (requires endoscopy) • Histology • Culture biopsy • Biopsy urease test (sometimes called CLO test) *Non-invasive* • Serology • Carbon-labelled urea breath test

Table 6(b) A comparison of available tests for detecting *H. pylori*. The accuracy and reliability of tests do have to be determined locally in use. The cost indications give a rough comparison between about £5 and £60 per test. Very many factors affect costs, especially availability of personnel to carry out the tests, and need for endoscopy.

Test	Sensitivity & specificity (approx.)	Cost range	Details
Histology	Both around 90–95%	£££	Needs local expertise Arguably a 'gold standard'
Biopsy and culture	Both around 90–95%	££	Needs local expertise Allows testing of antibiotic sensitivities Another 'gold standard'
Biopsy urease test	90–95%	£	Gives rapid results
Serology	85–95%	£	Not all tests have been widely validated Probably useful for screening dyspeptic patients for investigations Not of practical value to assess treatment success
Carbon-labelled urea breath tests	Both around 95%	££	Needs test kits ^{13}C can be carried out at a 'distance' [14]C cannot be used in children or pregnant women Neither reliable after gastric surgery Probably most useful test to evaluate success of treatment

identify them on standard haematoxylin and eosin stained sections. Technically, these stains do not prove the organism seen to be *H. pylori*, this can only be done using specific immunostaining or perhaps even the polymerase chain reaction. These techniques are rarely used in clinical situations and are reserved for research studies. In practice, the only confusion likely to arise is with the appearance of an unrelated but similar-looking organism, at present called *H. heilmanni* (previously *Gastrospirillum hominis*), which is rarely (<1% of cases) associated with chronic active gastritis similar to that caused by *H. pylori*. In general, however, histological investigation of *H. pylori* is both a highly specific and sensitive test (both around 90–95%) for *H. pylori* infection of the gastric antrum. Organisms tend to be harder to detect in surgical excision specimens than biopsy samples but, usually, at least two antral biopsies are necessary. Overall, histology is moderately expensive, being largely labour-intensive and, of course, also taking time and with the additional expense and necessity of a prior endoscopic procedure.

Another similar organism

Is histology the gold standard?

Bacteriological culture

Originally, *H. pylori* was regarded as a difficult organism to grow. This was because growth is slow and it is an anaerobic organism. The first isolation has now become legendary, growth having occurred because plates were left longer than normal over a holiday weekend.

For the best chances of culturing *H. pylori*, samples should be placed in medium as quickly as possible. *H. pylori* is, paradoxically, quickly killed in gastric juice acid. It presumably only survives in the stomach in the protected environment below the gastric mucus layer adjacent to gastric epithelial cells. Perhaps a neutral pH is maintained in this situation from the production of ammonia by the action of the organism's urease enzyme on endogenous urea. *H. pylori* is also intolerant of bile salts, which are present in the stomach of some individuals. In fact, it seems fairly strange that the organism can survive in the stomach at all!

Samples should be maintained in broth or saline if there is likely to be a delay getting them to the bacteriology laboratory. This should prevent the organism drying out and limits the oxygen concentration in the local environment. *H. pylori* has been found to survive much better if the temperature is kept low, and at about 4°C (refrigerator temperature) it will survive for hours if not days at a time. The

H. *pylori* in culture

Transporting it to the laboratory

organism can also be kept more or less indefinitely deep-frozen at −70°C. Once in the laboratory, best results are obtained by grinding or mincing biopsies. The organism is most ideally grown on agar plates including blood and selective antibiotics to prevent growth of other micro-organisms. Cultures need to be moist and in an atmosphere of only 5% oxygen, and will usually grow at a temperature of 37°C. Bacteria normally take at least 2–3 days to appear and sometimes are not apparent for 6–7 days. The colonies are usually small, often transparent or greyish but, on some media, may be tan coloured and the colour can be enhanced by addition of stains to the medium. Best recovery rates are from biopsies but the organism can be cultured from fresh gastric juice. In undesirable growth conditions *H. pylori*, as do some *Campylobacter* organisms, loses the typical spiral appearance and becomes the so-called 'coccoid' form. In this state the organism can exist for prolonged periods of time in an apparently viable condition.

Growing the organism

Organisms may be recognized for research purposes by immunoblot fingerprinting and restriction endonuclease DNA analysis. However, some individuals have been shown to have more than one type of bacteria within the stomach at any one time, and so it is unclear as to how relevant these techniques really are.

Bacteriological culture is a highly sensitive and specific test (both around 90–95%) but requires local expertise. Individual cultures are not expensive but, once again, the procedure is fairly labour-intensive. It has the advantage of permitting concurrent testing of antibiotic sensitivities. This is probably most useful against metronidazole in clinical practice but, in some populations, it may also be relevant to include sensitivity tests to clarithromycin.

How good is bacteriology?

3.1.2 Indirect tests

H. pylori possesses a number of enzymes but one that has created great interest is urease. This particular enzyme is produced in large amounts and is thought to be present on the surface of the organism. The main interest in this is the ability of the enzyme to convert endogenous urea, widely present in body fluids, to ammonia and release carbon

The urease enzyme

dioxide. Although this may have significance in relation to the pathogenesis of *H. pylori*-related gastroduodenal damage, it is also the basis of a number of indirect tests for the detection of this organism.

The presence of urease activity in mammalian gastric mucosa has been recognized for the best part of this century, but only in recent years has the source been identified as *H. pylori*. It is possible that the urease enzyme can be inhibited by omeprazole treatment. Whether this can upset urease-based tests is uncertain, but it should possibly be borne in mind.

Biopsy urease test

CLO testing

This test is based upon the principles previously outlined (Figs 15 & 16). A gastric mucosal biopsy, usually taken at endoscopy, is placed in a urea broth or on agar gel. Growth of the organism is not required, and the test relies on the presence of pre-formed urease enzyme. No other organism present in gastric mucosal biopsies, apart from *H. pylori*, would be expected to be urease producers in normal circumstances. When ammonia is formed in the medium, the subsequent pH change can be recognized by the use of a suitable indicator solution. Usually phenol red is used, and the colour changes from a yellow–brown to pink. Various commercial test systems exist, but the fastest can give a

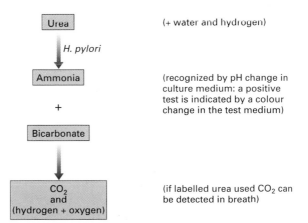

Fig. 15 How the urease test works.

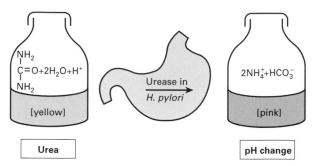

Fig. 16 Principle of the biopsy urease test.

positive reaction within an hour. Some will work at room temperature, but others are best if incubated at 37°C.

The cheapest and easiest of tests

The main advantage of the urease test is its cheapness, and it has to be one of the most competitively priced of all *H. pylori* detection methods. It is, however, less sensitive and specific than direct tests (although most should give results >90%). The test requires no specific skills to carry it out, and only basic levels of equipment are necessary. The results are usually obtained fairly rapidly, with most commercially available systems.

Urea breath test

Labelled urea breath testing

Urease activity is similarly the basis of urea breath tests, but this time it is the production of CO_2 from urea rather than ammonia release which is important. Urea is labelled at the carbon atom with either the stable non-radioactive isotope ^{13}C or weakly radioactive [14]C. This labelled compound is given in the form of a test meal and the labelled carbon is transferred to CO_2 under the influence of urease enzyme in the stomach. Labelled CO_2 enters the bloodstream, is excreted by the lungs and can be detected in a breath sample by an appropriate method. [14]C can be measured using a normal scintillation counter available in most hospitals but, being radioactive, has to be closely monitored. [13]C, on the other hand, whilst being perfectly safe, requires specific measurement with a mass spectrometer, only available in a few but increasing number of centres (Fig. 17).

The breath test itself

Patients undergoing this test usually fast overnight and are then given a fat-containing liquid test meal of several

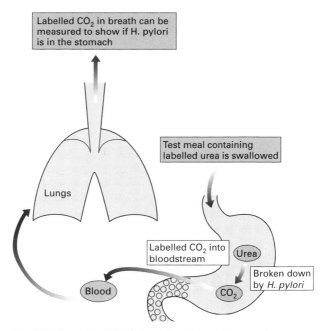

Fig. 17 The carbon-labelled urea breath test. A test meal containing a 'label' is given to the person to drink (the label is tied to urea). In the stomach, *H. pylori* has an enzyme which can digest urea and release labelled CO_2 into the bloodstream. This travels to the lungs and is breathed out. It can be measured in the breath sample to show *H. pylori* is in the stomach.

hundred millilitres volume (the fat delays gastric empty-ing). Breath samples are then collected at intervals for 2 hours or so, although some test systems only require a single breath sample, exhaled breath being blown into a solution that will trap the CO_2. Urease breath tests are extremely accurate and reliable (about 95%) and ^{14}C is re-latively cheap once the test has been set up. [13]C requires special facilities and costs are moderately expensive. The breath test is not reliable in someone who has had previous gastric surgery. [14]C, being radioactive, is not suitable for pregnant women or young children. Probably the main place for using breath tests is in assessing the effects of treatment when patients can be tested a minimum of

Breath tests to monitor treatment

4 weeks after completing a course of therapy aimed at eradicating *H. pylori*. ^{13}C breath tests can be carried out at 'a distance' by using the postal service.

Serological tests

As with most bacterial infections, *H. pylori* stimulates an immune response and circulating antibodies appear in the peripheral bloodstream. This is the basis for serology tests to diagnose *H. pylori* infection.

In acute infection, which is uncommonly seen, IgM levels are raised but these fall with time, so that in the long term both IgG and IgA levels to *H. pylori* are elevated.

Serum antibodies

Antibodies can be measured in a number of different ways, but most tests use an enzyme-linked immunosorbent assay (ELISA). In this test, *H. pylori* antigen is suspended onto a plastic microtitre plate and washed. Human immunoglobulin bound to this (from the serum sample being tested) is measured using an antibody made against this immunoglobulin, which also has an attached label. The marker usually used is an enzyme (most commonly peroxidase) and this can be visualized by adding a coloured substrate and the amount binding can be measured in a light-sensitive meter. The optical density of this coloured product is thus proportional to the amount of bound antibody.

Western blotting techniques can also be carried out to determine antibody responses to specific antigenic components, but this is usually of value only in research experiments.

Commercial tests need validating

Serology is now a highly sensitive and specific test (85–95%) for current or past *H. pylori* infection. Originally, serology was limited to specific laboratories, but now a range of commercially available test kits for use on both peripheral blood and some also for saliva samples have been introduced. The major problem with these is that not all have been validated against accepted means of diagnosing *H. pylori* infection and generally they appear somewhat difficult to use in practice and are less reliable than tests based upon serum samples. Cross-reaction with *Campylobacter* is one problem that can be countered by absorption with appropriate antigens, but it is not always clear with the commercial kits that this has been done. Usually only one antigen preparation has been used to prepare reagents and that organism may not be relevant to different populations in other countries to the place where the test was developed. The surface antigenic material used is often, in fact, the urease antigen. Most serological tests should be moderately priced and relatively easy to carry out without necessarily having considerable background knowledge and skill. There is some evidence that titre ranges may be different in children and adults.

Serology best for deciding which dyspeptics to investigate

Serology is an ideal tool for epidemiological investigations. Perhaps its major use in clinical practice is to aid in the evaluation of patients with dyspepsia. Because of the close links between *H. pylori* and conditions associated with dyspepsia, including peptic ulcer disease and possibly gastric cancer, it has been suggested that, along with older dyspeptics (those >45 years of age) and those patients with dyspepsia receiving non-steroidal anti-inflammatory drugs (NSAIDs), endoscopy should also include those positive for *H. pylori*. This approach has been shown to reliably pick up most of those with dyspepsia having 'significant' underlying disease such as ulcers and gastric cancer, yet reduce endoscopic workload by about one-quarter. Serology is, however, of little use in monitoring the effects of *H. pylori* eradication treatment. Antibody levels take too long to fall (often several months) to be a reliable determinant.

3.2 Treating H. pylori infection

Clearance and eradication

A range of treatments can influence *H. pylori* infection and produce temporary suppression and apparent *clearance* of the organism. This is thus defined as the absence of *H. pylori* for up to 4 weeks after treatment has stopped. Inadequate treatment can therefore result in a flare-up and reappearance of infection or recrudescence. Permanent *eradication*, on the other hand, is defined as the absence of *H. pylori* infection more than 4 weeks after treatment has finished. Omeprazole, for instance, appears to have a direct effect on the organism, as does bismuth, to suppress growth but permanent eradication is unusual when either agent is used alone.

Many agents work *in vitro*

Most of the available treatments were initially evaluated in *in vitro* laboratory tests, but these do not necessarily truly reflect the situation when infection is established on gastric mucosa. For instance, in culture, the sugar-rich outer protective layer, or glycocalyx, of *H. pylori* is much thinner than that observed in real life and this may affect antibacterial penetration. Furthermore, in the intact stomach, gastric acid may well have a deleterious effect on antibiotic bioavailability. The location of *H. pylori* during infection in the antrum of the stomach, with some possibly in the fundus in severe infections, lying deep in gastric pits, may make access to drugs used in treatment very limited. It is still not clear whether treatment should be aimed at achieving high concentrations of antibiotics in the stomach lumen or absorption and subsequent excretion of these drugs into the stomach through the gastric mucosa.

3.2.1 Monotherapy

In vitro effects

Single therapy treatment

In culture, *H. pylori* is extremely sensitive to a range of penicillins, cephalosporins, tetracyclines, macrolides, including erythromycin and clarithromycin and the quinolones. Metronidazole has modest activity but its use is restricted by the resistance of a number of strains. In most European studies, the resistance rates are about 20–40% of those examined, but in some Asian communities in the UK 90% or more of strains have been found resistant. Macrolide resistance, particularly to clarithromycin, appears to exist in some (affecting 10% of certain populations) but is not a problem in all localities. In general, most ulcer-healing drugs have little laboratory activity against *H. pylori*, bismuth and the proton-pump inhibitors being exceptions. Omeprazole and bismuth have modest *in vitro* activity but lansoprozole appears to have more marked properties in this regard which extend to its principal active metabolites. The clinical trial work with this compound against *H. pylori*, to date, does not appear to particularly mirror the *in vitro* efficacy and overall it appears about as effective as omeprazole. Pantoprazole is the next proton-pump inhibitor to come onto the market but few significant studies have been carried out with this agent in relation to *H. pylori* infection.

Antibiotic resistance is a problem

Bismuth

Although bismuth compounds have significant effects on laboratory cultures, the responses have not been very good when used alone in patients. Bismuth is, however, interesting since it attains anti-*H. pylori* activity at levels which can be achieved in the gastric mucosa. Bismuth inhibits the urease activity of the organism and can cause rapid detachment of bacteria from the gastric epithelial cells and death of the bacteria since these are quickly coated by bismuth salts. Of course, bismuth has been used for years for dyspeptic symptoms, firstly as Roter tablets and more recently, particularly in the United States, as the subsalicylate in the form of PeptoBismol. It is speculative that its effects on symptoms were by having an anti-*Helicobacter* activity. It is perhaps of interest to recall that injections of bismuth were used for treating that other well-known spirochaete *Treponema pallidum* in the pre-penicillin era. One of the main attractions of bismuth salts is the lack of toxicity in the absence of renal impairment, apart from darkening of the stools. However, bismuth encephalopathy has been recorded in the past when extremely high dosages have been given — much more than would be used for *Helicobacter* treatment. It should not, however, be used except for fixed lengths of treatment. One of the other benefits of bismuth salts is that they appear to have mucosal healing effects, apparently independent of any action against *H. pylori,* and courses produce excellent healing rates for peptic ulcers.

Bismuth has been used for many years to treat dyspepsia

Bismuth has a mucosal healing effect

Urease inhibitors

Another approach that has been tried to tackle *H. pylori* infection is to inhibit the actions of urease, since this appears to be an important 'virulence' factor. There are not many urease inhibitors to choose from and several are toxic. Some attempts have been made using acetohydroxamic acid, without any great success.

Urease inhibitors probably do not work

Antibiotic monotherapy

Clarithromycin appears best

Other single agents are generally ineffective for various reasons. Clarithromycin is one of the best but erythromycin is unstable in the acidic conditions of the normal stomach (Table 7). Quinolones, another group with marked effects against cultured *H. pylori*, are of no value in clinical usage because of the rapid development of antibiotic resistance by the organism. Fortunately, these problems do not appear to affect amoxycillin or ampicillin, which are less affected by gastric pH, and resistance is not a practical problem to date. Metronidazole and tinidazole are similarly apparently unaffected by pH, but acquired resistance is a problem unless they are given in combination with probably at least two other bactericidal drugs (Table 8). Use of metronidazole has been limited by the metallic taste left in the mouth, nausea, diarrhoea, furring of the tongue and other severe side-effects if taken in combination with alcohol (disulfiram-like side-effects). A number of suggestions have been made about the ideal means of administering various drugs and when they should be taken in relation to food, but no clear-cut pattern has emerged although most appear to work better the more frequently they are given.

Many single antibiotics are not effective

Metronidazole has side-effects

Table 7 Antibiotic treatment—clarithromycin.

- One of the most active treatments against *H. pylori*
- Primary resistance much lower than with metronidazole, but more expensive and resistance can develop
- Associated with a low frequency of side-effects
- Useful alternative in patients with penicillin allergy or previous treatment failure

Table 8 *H. pylori*: antimicrobial resistance in the UK.

Resistance	Median (%)	Range
Metronidazole*	39	15–65
Tinidazole	28	7–42
Clarithromycin	5	1–13

* Resistance is higher in: (i) inner cities (vs. rural areas); (ii) people <40 years; and (iii) women.

Acid suppressants

Proton-pump inhibitors suppress growth

Antacids may have limited effects when given to patients with gastritis, in that some studies have suggested a diminution in *H. pylori* densities, but not all have agreed. In general, acid suppressants alone have only mild, if any, effects on *H. pylori* in patients. The H_2 receptor antagonists appear to lack efficacy, but omeprazole and lansoprazole may have some. Certainly in laboratory cultures, omeprazole has *in vitro* effects at reasonably low doses. Lansoprazole appears even more effective and so do its active breakdown products. There is increasing published evidence using lansoprazole against *H. pylori* infection. At the current time, in dual and triple therapy combinations it appears about as effective as omeprazole. In patients, sole use of omeprazole appears to have some influence by suppressing growth of the bacterium, particularly in the antrum, but may leave organisms elsewhere, and particularly higher in the stomach in the fundus, relatively unaffected. There is also some *in vitro* evidence that omeprazole itself rather than its active metabolites may affect *H. pylori* bacterial urease. Whether this has any clinical effects is totally uncertain, but it may interfere with non-invasive tests for *H. pylori* dependent on urease activity, such as the carbon-labelled urea breath tests. Apart from bismuth, no other ulcer-healing drugs otherwise have dramatic effects on *H. pylori* infection.

Honey

Honey may work!

One other interesting observation made in laboratory cultures is the use of honey. This, like bismuth, has been used for years by patients for indigestion symptoms. A certain type has been shown to have effects in the laboratory against *H. pylori*—but it has to be a variety from New Zealand!

Overall, unfortunately, no single agent gives reliable results in the eradication of *H. pylori* from patients. As such, monotherapy for eradication of this organism cannot be recommended since, if it does anything at all, depending on what is used, it is likely to cause side-effects, have limited clinical benefits and may induce bacterial resistance to that agent in the community at large.

3.2.2 Dual therapy

The older dual therapies were not generally bactericidal

Dual therapy has been widely used in an attempt to produce *H. pylori* eradication. In general, however, it appears that, until recently, most dual therapy regimens available were not bactericidal against *H. pylori*. Although many combinations have been tried, most experience has been reported with bismuth, omeprazole, lansoprazole or ranitidine bismuth citrate in combination with an antibacterial, most commonly amoxycillin/clarithromycin or metronidazole/tinidazole.

Bismuth and metronidazole

Using two drugs only appears to increase antibiotic resistance

In general, efficacy with bismuth and metronidazole is probably one of the most consistent dual therapy regimens, with eradication rates of up to 75% having been achieved. Unfortunately, resistance of the organism has also been reported to occur during treatment with bismuth and metronidazole and, therefore, this type of regimen should not now be used.

Omeprazole and amoxycillin

Omeprazole and antibiotics

A very large number of studies has been carried out using a dual combination of omeprazole and amoxycillin, with widely differing eradication rates varying from 0 to 93%. In general, the higher doses appear to offer best results (at least 40 mg omeprazole daily). The majority of these studies have involved small numbers of patients (often 20–30 in total, some with many less) and few have been published in substantive journal reports. One large study involved 157 patients and achieved an eradication rate of 54%, which is approximately the mean result of all the other available studies. Although a licence has been granted for this combination in the UK, results are unacceptable for routine clinical usage in attempting to eradicate *H. pylori* and this combination should therefore no longer be used. Furthermore, extremely limited data exist with this combination when used in peptic ulcer disease that confirm reduced ulcer recurrence rates.

Omeprazole and clarithromycin

Because of these problems, more recently omeprazole, lamsoprazole and ranitidine bismuth citrate have been combined with clarithromycin and similar principles seem to apply. Overall eradication rates appear somewhat more encouraging (between about 46 and 82%), higher doses of omeprazole are most effective and the optimum dose of clarithromycin appears to be 1.5 g/day, but some trials published to date involve small patient numbers, few have been formally published and these combinations are expensive.

There appear to be more effective dual therapies

Overall, although dual therapy regimens have suddenly become very popular and are currently being widely prescribed, their use, except for those including clarithromycin, is not supported by proven efficacy in inducing *H. pylori* eradication. Furthermore, long-term follow-up of treated patients has, as yet, shown extremely limited clinical benefits, if any.

3.2.3 Triple therapy

Triple therapy is very good overall

The general disappointment with the results obtained using both single and most dual therapy regimens against *H. pylori* has focused attention mainly on the use of triple therapies.

Bismuth triple therapy

The original experience with triple therapy was with combinations including bismuth, usually together with two antibacterials, namely amoxycillin or tetracycline and metronidazole, or tinidazole. Although many refer to 'bismuth triple therapy', there is little consensus on the dosages used or the duration of treatment that should be given. Published eradication rates fall in the range of about 55–95% of patients treated, but, in practice, many achieve results only towards the lower end of those reported. Overall, most would agree that combinations including

Regimens with tetracycline give better results

√√√

tetracycline give marginally better results than those with amoxycillin, but the differences are probably not terribly significant. Most of the drugs have to be taken three to four times each day for best results, and this may influence compliance. This is probably also very much affected by the incidence of side-effects, which is often fairly considerable (Table 9). Studies have suggested that about one-fifth of patients taking this treatment have to discontinue it before completion because of side-effects—many of these actively causing gastrointestinal symptoms including nausea, vomiting and diarrhoea! The other limiting factor to this regimen is the incidence of metronidazole resistance, which means therapy is probably ineffective anyway in about one-quarter to one-third of most patient groups (see Table 10). For these reasons such combinations have little if any place as first-line treatment nowadays.

Acid-suppressant triple therapy

The limitations of bismuth triple therapy have led to the development of acid-suppressant triple therapy regimens. These are a combination of either omeprazole, lansoprazole or ranitidine bismuth citrate or ranitidine with antibacterials, usually either amoxycillin, tetracycline or clarithromycin with metronidazole or tinidazole. A large number of studies have now been carried out with these regimens, and some of the published data are excellent and produce eradication reproducibly in around 85% of patients taking 7 days of treatment. Side-effects appear relatively sparse (probably around 10% of patients or less) and although compliance difficulties probably remain a problem because of the number of tablets or capsules required, duration of necessary treatment is being reduced and failure rates due to side-effects also appear to be falling. Antibiotic resistance remains a problem with some of the

Low side-effects, but compliance may be a problem

Table 9 Triple eradication therapy—major problems.

- Side-effects of antibiotics (largely gastrointestinal)
- Interactions (especially alcohol and nitroimidazoles)
- Antibacterial resistance (metronidazole in particular)
- Patient compliance (multiple drugs)

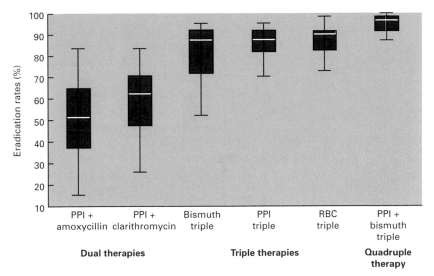

Fig. 18 Comparison of the *H. pylori* eradication treatments. PPI, proton pump inhibitor; RBC, ranitidine bismuth citrate.

Acid-suppressant triple therapies give optimum clinical results ✓✓

drugs. However, in routine clinical practice these combinations probably give nearest to optimal results. Most acid-suppressant triple therapies given on an 'intention to treat' basis achieve eradication rates of over 80%, which is now generally regarded as ideal (Fig. 18).

3.2.4 Quadruple therapy

Quadruple therapy appears best so far! ✓✓

The combination of acid-suppressant triple therapy together with colloidal bismuth has been used as quadruple therapy. This arguably gives the best overall results for *H. pylori* eradication (about 93–98%). In three trials in which this combination was compared with standard triple therapy, the quadruple treatment was significantly better in two.

3.2.5 Ranitidine bismuth citrate

Ranitidine bismuth citrate is a new entity

It appears that it may be possible to provide the benefits of triple therapy but in a dual treatment regimen. Ranitidine bismuth citrate has been developed not as a mixture of two previously successful drugs, but as a new molecular complex, which is a discrete chemical entity. It is the first compound developed specifically to have anti-*Helicobacter* activity. It has a number of unique properties, appearing to combine antisecretory, pepsin inhibition, mucosal protection and anti-*H. pylori* effects. Although when used alone in clinical trials it has limited efficacy in inducing eradication, in combination with clarithromycin it appears to achieve similar eradication rates to those obtained with many triple therapies (around 85+%). Ranitidine bismuth citrate is also effective in triple therapy combinations with two antibacterials, usually either amoxycillin and clarithromycin or clarithromycin and tinidazole/metronidazole. In 7-day treatment courses eradication success has been reported on an 'intention to treat' basis of between 83% and 88%.

Ranitidine bismuth citrate plus clarithromycin — results are encouraging

Table 10 Current limitations to *H. pylori* eradication.

- Compliance; especially with triple therapy
- Side-effects of treatment; means 20% of patients on some regimens fail to complete the course
- Resistance to antibacterials; particularly metronidazole — 20–40% of many populations resistant
- Recurrence or recrudescence of inadequately treated infection; rates are not entirely certain but with current triple therapy regimens are probably small

3.2.6 Eradication or suppression?

One problem associated with current treatment not mentioned so far is the problem of achieving a permanent 'cure' of *H. pylori* after eradication has been achieved. Reported results vary widely in differing studies and using different techniques, and range from 1.2% recurrence in the West to 9% per year in developing countries. Some of the higher figures may be due to inadequate initial 'eradication' treatment. There is evidence to suggest that some omeprazole regimens simply produce suppression of growth and perhaps not true eradication with subsequent recrudescence of this inadequately treated infection. This potentially introduces practical problems in treatment. Preferably, proton-pump inhibitor pre-treatment is prob-

Re-infection and recrudescence of infection

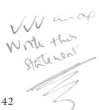

ably best stopped for a couple of weeks at least before giving *H. pylori* eradication therapy, although not all agree this is necessary. Nevertheless, there is a whole range of reported 're-infection' rates in between these extremes and no doubt we will have to wait to find out the true risks in our own clinical practices. Although adequate data are currently unavailable, it is widely believed at present that if infection is adequately treated initially, the risk of re-infection occurring in the short term, up to about 1 year and probably also beyond, in Western countries, is low — probably only 1 or 2% per year. However, until we are certain how and where re-infection comes from, we are unlikely to fully understand the problems of recurrent infection after *H. pylori* eradication treatment.

3.3 Who should receive H. pylori treatment?

Not for everyone!

Although *H. pylori* has been described in association with a number of clinical conditions, there are currently relatively few situations where eradication treatment is indicated. With an infective process affecting up to half of many population groups, it is obviously essential to have strictly defined criteria for attempting *H. pylori* eradication (see Fig. 19). Furthermore, because of the inadequacies of many existing treatment regimens and the risks (albeit uncommon) of significant side-effects with some forms of therapy, adherence to specific indications for treatment is of paramount importance.

The 'expert' opinions

Various groups of individuals with interest in this field have met, often on an *ad hoc* basis, to attempt to define treatment aims and indications. These were firstly on an international level but now protocols and recommendations are filtering down to both national and local levels. One of the earliest was a working party associated with the World Congresses of Gastroenterology, which met in 1990. Although much has changed in our treatment approaches since this time, some of their conclusions remain valid today. This group recommended restricting treatment to patients with duodenal ulcer (DU) disease and not attempting therapy in those with non-ulcer dyspepsia (NUD) or those with gastric ulcers since they felt there was insufficient evidence to justify this. Furthermore, they suggested that:

> . . . for the time being *H. pylori* therapy should be reserved for those groups of patients where it has been shown unequivocally to have an advantage over the currently available cytoprotective and acid-suppressive drugs

> . . . in those individuals where DU is a serious management problem . . . or where complications . . . have occurred, *H. pylori* eradication should be attempted

> If *H. pylori* therapy is undertaken, the most effective treatment regimen should be employed.

They were, therefore, recommending the treatment of a relatively small group of DU patients with triple therapy, which, at the time, was essentially bismuth triple therapy.

The NIH consensus

These conclusions have been further considered and expanded more recently by a consensus group established by the prestigious National Institutes of Health (NIH) in the United States. Once again they recommended restricting treatment to those with peptic ulcer disease, specifically suggesting avoiding attempts in those with NUD or those patients with a potential risk of gastric cancer (Table 11).

Limited evidence that *H. pylori* eradication reduces ulcer complications

They did not feel confident enough to advise reliance on *H. pylori* eradication as a means of preventing long-term ulcer complications such as bleeding or perforation. Although some evidence does exist to suggest that *H. pylori* eradication treatment reduces the risk of re-bleeding in peptic ulcer patients who have had an episode of haemorrhage, the studies that have been published

Table 11 NIH consensus statement.

- Ulcer patients with *H. pylori* infection require antimicrobial and antisecretory drugs (Maintenance acid suppression may also be wise in those who have suffered a bleeding ulcer)
- Value of treating *H. pylori* in non-ulcer dyspepsia remains uncertain
- The relationship between *H. pylori* and gastric cancer requires further exploration

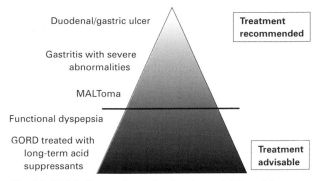

Fig. 19 Which diseases for eradication therapy? Adapted from The Maastricht Consensus Report.

involve small numbers of patients followed only for short periods of time. There is, however, little specific reason to believe *H. pylori* eradication would reduce these risks, since current evidence suggests that perforated ulcer patients, and possibly those having had an ulcer bleed, are no more likely than age-matched normal individuals to be positive for *H. pylori* infection. Epidemiological studies suggest that use of NSAIDs are particularly linked to inducing peptic ulcer complications. Currently it is generally accepted that maintenance treatment with long-term acid suppression (mainly shown for the H_2 receptor antagonists cimetidine and ranitidine) is the best way to reduce bleeding or perforation of ulcers—reducing the risks of haemorrhage, for instance, from probably more than 10% of patients over a 5-year period to 1–2% of patients during a similar period of time. Concurrent treatment in NSAID users with omeprazole or an H_2 receptor antagonist may also be helpful long term in reducing bleeding risks.

The overall conclusions of the NIH group were that 'ulcer patients with *H. pylori* infection require treatment with antimicrobial agents in addition to antisecretory drugs whether on first presentation with the illness or on recurrence' (Fig. 19).

Treat ulcer patients for *H.pylori*

In practice, if the patient is in the normal adult age-range and presents with an uncomplicated DU, there is little to be gained by checking *H. pylori* status since, invariably, most of these patients will be positive. Outside these age-ranges, and for patients with gastric ulceration (GU), that is

Up to date
guidance from
around the world

less certain since, particularly in GU disease, NSAID ingestion is more frequently the provocative or causative factor.

In 1997, three consensus reports appeared more or less
synchronously in the United States (The Digestive Health
Initiative formed by The American Digestive Health Foundation), in Europe (The Maastricht Consensus Report
from the European *Helicobacter pylori* Study Group) and
the Asia Pacific region (Asia Pacific Consensus Confer-
ences). They all broadly support and extend the indications
for *H. pylori* eradication identified in previous consensus
statements.

In the American opinion, testing and treatment should
take place for patients with an active or documented past
history of duodenal ulcer, gastric ulcer and complicated
duodenal or gastric ulcer, for those who have had a resec-
tion of early gastric cancer or low-grade gastric mucosa-
associated lymphoid tissue (MALT) lymphoma but not for
patients with undiagnosed dyspeptic symptoms.

The European view was broadly similar although adding
that treatment was 'advisable' or 'strongly recommended'
with either 'unequivocal or supportive' evidence for those
with gastritis and severe abnormalities, those with
oesophageal reflux disease treated by long-term proton-
pump inhibitors and after surgery for peptic ulcer disease.
Many of these latter categories could be questioned on the
basis of existing evidence (Fig. 19).

The Asia Pacific consensus document was somewhat
broader including for testing and/or treatment those with
previous peptic ulceration or a history of dyspepsia due to
be started on NSAIDs, those with dyspepsia who were
found to be *H. pylori* positive, perhaps those with a family
history of gastric cancer since this is a so common in the Far
East, and those who ask to be tested for *H. pylori*, accepting
that evidence for benefit in some if not all these latter categories is lacking.

Managing dyspeptic conditions in the H. pylori era

Ulcer causes are multi-factorial

Despite the discovery of *H. pylori*, it is still widely accepted by most working in the field that peptic ulceration remains a disease with many factors playing a causative role. Acid, and perhaps pepsin and bicarbonate secretion, bile reflux, cigarette smoking, consumption of aspirin and other non-steroidal anti-inflammatory drugs (NSAIDs), genetic and possibly also some other environmental factors apart from those already mentioned, appear important in at least some, if not all, patients (Table 12).

The pathogenesis of non-ulcer dyspepsia (NUD) is generally extremely poorly understood (Fig. 20). There is evidence to incriminate acid secretion in some, perhaps a motility disturbance in others and psychosocial factors may also sometimes be important. Nevertheless, *H. pylori* infection remains particularly prevalent in this population overall, yet its role is far from clear. Reflux oesophagitis is arguably the commonest of all dyspeptic conditions in which undoubtedly acid and bile reflux and primary motility disturbances play a part, and yet, in the light of current evidence, *H. pylori* has no direct role in this disorder whatsoever. There is in fact some indirect evidence that *H. pylori* infection of the stomach may offer some protection against gastro-oesophageal reflux disease.

Other factors cause reflux disease

The importance of *H. pylori* in dyspeptic conditions is certain, but it is perhaps too early to conclude that discovery of this organism should completely revolutionize our management of all patients suffering from upper gut symptoms.

With regard to *H. pylori* eradication in the management of dyspepsia, diagnosis of the underlying condition is the first essential stage (Table 13). It is generally accepted that patients presenting with dyspepsia for the first time over the age of about 45–50 years should be investigated, either by endoscopy or barium meal, depending on which is the most readily available and reliable in an individual geo-

First diagnose the dyspeptics

Table 12 Causative factors in peptic ulceration.

Acid + pepsin	'No acid, no ulcer'
Bacteria	*H. pylori*
Cigarettes	Heavy smokers have lower healing rates and higher recurrence rates
Drugs	Especially salicylates and NSAIDs
Environment	?? stress- or diet-related factors
Family history	DU patients often have first-degree relatives with ulcer disease; also blood group related

Table 13 Which dyspeptic patient should be investigated?

- 45 years old or greater at first presentation
- Those who relapse as soon as treatment stopped or who never responded
- Those on NSAIDs
- Those who are *H. pylori* positive

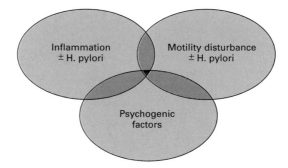

Fig. 20 Likely pathogenesis of non-ulcer dyspepsia.

graphic area (Table 14). Others who should be included for investigation are those taking NSAIDs or have other worrying features, such as anorexia, weight loss, persistent symptoms despite treatment, associated significant vomiting or abdominal mass (Tables 15 & 16).

Treating the dyspeptic

The remainder can largely be safely treated initially with an antacid, with or without an acid suppressant such as an H_2 receptor antagonist (H_2RA), cimetidine or ranitidine

Table 14 Endoscopy or barium radiology.*

Endoscopy	Radiology
Usually preferred for: • known gastric ulcers • suspected or previously known duodenal ulcer • suspected carcinoma • previous gastric surgery • elderly or immobile patients • detection of mucosal inflammatory disease • diagnosis of active *H. pylori* infection • testing bacterial sensitivities in association with anti-*H. pylori* treatment	Usually preferred for: • dysphagia, especially if proximal (high) • suspected oesophageal motility disorder (non-cardiac chest pain)

* There are some situations in which one investigation is preferred over the other. If in doubt, discuss with your local gastroenterologist/radiologist.

Table 15 Indications for referral or investigation of the upper GI tract.

• Dyspepsia (see Table 13) • Dysphagia (radiology arguably better if symptoms are 'high') • Unexplained iron-deficiency anaemia/weight loss • Haematemesis/melaena (usually urgent) • Persistent undiagnosed symptoms and signs if barium radiology is negative

for a 4- to 6 week course (Table 17). Reflux-type dyspepsia can be reasonably accurately diagnosed clinically. Most would agree that an antacid/alginate is appropriate first-line treatment for most of these patients followed if necessary by a course of proton-pump inhibitor (PPI) if symptoms are severe or persistent. Any who fail to respond, or where symptoms continue or relapse as soon as treatment is discontinued, should then be considered for investigations. Those with access to *H. pylori* testing, either by serology or urea breath tests, may have a further discriminant for deciding who to investigate, limiting this to those over 45 years of age, those taking NSAIDs or who are *H. pylori* positive (see Table 13).

Those needing investigation

In general, patients who should otherwise be considered for further investigation are those with dyspepsia who have

49

Table 16 Selection guidelines for open-access upper GI endoscopy. Open-access endoscopy is the referral for endoscopy usually without a hospital consultation and a report on the procedure returned directly to the referring doctor.

General indications

Dyspeptic patients
- all patients >45 years of age with a short history
- those with a previously normal barium meal, diagnostic/management problems and those in whom a negative result is likely to be helpful (especially patients taking NSAIDs/failed acid-suppressive treatment or relapse once treatment stopped)
- those requiring tissue diagnosis, especially gastric ulcer or suspected malignancy/Barrett's oesophagus/*H. pylori* antibiotic sensitivities

Main contra-indications to open-access endoscopy

Relative exclusions
- very severe cardiac/respiratory disease, including rheumatic heart disease and patients with recent myocardial infarction/unstable angina
- significant other concurrent disease
- severe rheumatoid disease with neck involvement
- proximal dysphagia
- sensitivity to benzodiazepines/anaesthetics
If there is doubt, the endoscopist should be consulted, especially if the patient is on anticoagulants, has diabetes or is pregnant

Requirements for endoscopy

Condensed medical history
- past medical history
- current drug treatment
- known drug reactions
Withhold ulcer-healing drug treatment if at all possible

Be aware that after sedation patients should not drive, operate machinery or be entirely self-reliant for 24 hours

Be aware that referral for endoscopy alone does not usually imply a clinical assessment nor that clinical responsibility, beyond undertaking the investigation, has been accepted

Rapid hospital referral

previously had normal upper gastrointestinal (GI) radiology, those shown to have gastric ulceration (GU), which must always be biopsied, or for any other specific indications such as dysphagia, haematemesis or melaena, weight loss thought to have a primarily upper GI cause and those with jaundice. Most of these latter categories would normally require *urgent* referral for hospital management rather than elective out-patient investigation (Table 18).

Table 17 Suggested management of the patient presenting with dyspepsia. Dyspepsia is an extremely common, loosely defined symptom complex. Most likely due to *reflux aesophagitis* (gastro-oesophageal reflux disease — GORD), *peptic ulceration* or *non-ulcer dyspepsia* (NUD). The main concern is that *gastric cancer*, albeit uncommon in the West, can present with dyspepsia. The risk of gastric cancer below 45 years of age is, however, small in much of Europe and the USA.

Patient	Action
>45 years of age or other worrying features, i.e. weight loss, anorexia, abdominal mass, first presentation at that age, etc.	Investigate • endoscopy or barium meal
<45 years of age, otherwise well	Treat • with antacid ± H$_2$RA for 6 weeks • If reflux-type dyspepsia, antacid/alginate ± PPI ± prokinetic Reassess • if well, no further action • continued symptoms or early relapse — endoscopy/barium meal
Persistent symptoms, endoscopy/barium meal negative	• If barium negative, consider endoscopy (investigations are complementary) • Consider other causes, e.g. gallstones, irritable bowel, etc. • Therefore: ultrasound, barium enema, etc. • Consider referral to gastroenterologist

H$_2$RA, H$_2$ receptor antagonist; PPI, proton-pump inhibitor.

Table 18 Rapid access gastrointestinal referrals. This is particularly indicated for patients with the conditions listed below.

- Dysphagia
- Suspicion of haematemesis/melaena (but not convincing enough to require immediate hospital admission)
- Recent significant change in bowel habit, particularly in those over the age of 40 years
- Significant rectal bleeding
- Marked anorexia/weight loss—thought to have a GI cause
- Persistent unremitting vomiting of more than a few days' duration
- Intractable abdominal pain
- Patients on NSAIDs developing GI symptoms
- Jaundice

4.1 Patients with peptic ulceration

Treating ulcers

Most would treat initially with an antacid and an acid suppressant—such as an H_2RA, cimetidine or ranitidine, or a PPI, omeprazole or lansoprazole or ranitidine bismuth citrate (RBC)—and give these in combination with two appropriate antibacterials, usually either amoxicillin or clarithromycin together with metronidazole or tinidazole

Table 19 Suggested management of known peptic ulcer disease.

Patient	Action
Symptomatic	Treat • antacid + H_2RA/proton-pump inhibitor/ranitidine bismuth citrate for 4–6 weeks (longer if GU) In addition in first 1–2 weeks give additional antibacterials as part of a recognized *H. pylori* eradication regimen. Supportive advice • stop smoking • avoid NSAIDs Check no complications • anaemia • if gastric ulcer, has biopsy been obtained? • subsequently confirm *H. pylori* eradication
Persistent symptoms or complications	Review diagnosis Consider referral to gastroenterologist
Those who are persistent management problems consider hospital assessment • GI bleeding/intractable pain	Urgent referral (usually requires admission)
• unresponsive symptoms • rapid recurrence of symptoms • young patients likely to need life-long maintenance	Routine referral

Attempted *H. pylori* eradication is indicated in patients with DU and also those with GU disease
Note that:
• eradication is *not* 100% successful
• there is a need to monitor eradication
• at least 20% of *H. pylori* are metronidazole resistant and suboptimal treatment will increase the risks of spreading resistance in the population
• drug treatment (such as triple therapy) is not without problems—expense, alcohol intolerance with metronidazole, GI disturbance, pseudomembranous colitis, etc.

for 1–2 weeks and advise lifestyle improvement, including stopping smoking and avoidance if possible of NSAIDs (Table 19). If the ulcer is active then some would continue the ulcer-healing agent for a further 4–6 weeks to ensure healing occurs. If the patient has a GU, it is most important to obtain biopsy material for histological examination and confirm healing after treatment. Any obvious complications suggesting GI bleeding or even perforation should be urgently referred for hospital management.

4.1.1 H. pylori eradication

H. pylori eradication in ulcers

H. pylori eradication should now be considered first-line treatment for all patients with duodenal ulceration (DU) and GU, although it is more controversial in those with ulcers thought to be NSAID induced. At present, it is probably inadvisable to manage patients who have experienced GI bleeding solely with attempts at *H. pylori* eradication.

Bleeding ulcers

These patients who are at high risk because they have had previous GI bleeding or perforation or who are elderly or have significant concurrent other medical diseases should perhaps also continue on long-term acid-suppression therapy (evidence rests largely with cimetidine or ranitidine) (Table 20). The evidence that *H. pylori* eradication is as effective in NSAID-induced ulceration is not as convincing as for DU and non-NSAID-induced GU disease. At present, attempts at eradication should not be

Table 20 Summary of guidelines for management of peptic ulcer.

Patient	Treatment
Any age, active or inactive ulcer	Acid suppressant or ulcer-healing agent plus antibacterials, 1–2 weeks
Recent complications (haemorrhage/perforation)	Heal ulcer and eradicate *H. pylori* (high-risk patients/elderly/ concurrent disease: consider long-term acid suppression as well)
NSAID user	Heal ulcer, not known whether *H. pylori* eradication advantageous in long term
Monitor results of treatment • often best done with carbon-labelled urea breath test, if available	

relied upon in these situations, although many would regard *H. pylori* eradication prudent (Tables 21 & 22). In NSAID-induced peptic ulceration, cimetidine, ranitidine and omeprazole are well established to promote healing, although probably only ranitidine, omeprazole and the prostaglandin analogue misoprostil have proven benefits in preventing ulcers and thus complications, including haem-

H. pylori appears to play a major role in the pathogenesis of duodenal and gastric ulcers

Eradication of *H. pylori*:

• Dramatically reduces the risk of DU recurrence and also that of GU disease

• Appears to modify the natural history of these diseases

Fig. 21 *H. pylori* and peptic ulceration.

Table 21 Suggested management of NSAID-induced ulcers.

Patient	Action
Symptomatic or recent GI bleed (excluding emergency treatment of bleeding)	Investigate • endoscopy usually best Treat • H$_2$RA or PPI 6–8 weeks stop, or consider change of NSAID • ? use 'pro-drug' or 'low-risk' NSAID
Previous GI complication of NSAID or 'high-risk' elderly patient, i.e. previous peptic ulcer, etc.	Consider concurrent H$_2$RA or PPI/prostaglandin analogue after successful *H. pylori* eradication has been achieved

Table 22 Who should have *H. pylori* treatment?

Duodenal ulcer Gastric ulcer	} · · · · · · · · · · · · · · · · Yes
Non-ulcer dyspepsia NSAID-induced ulcers	} · · · · · · · · · · · · · · · Possibly
Gastro-oesophageal reflux Concerns about stomach cancer	} · · · · · · · · · · · · · · · · No

orrhage. Alternative approaches are in trying to reduce or discontinue NSAID usage or use a different NSAID which may be anticipated to be less harmful (see Table 21).

Various regimens

Present opinion advocates the incorporation during the first 1–2 weeks of the healing regimen of an acid suppressant such as ranitidine, omeprazole or lansoprazole or RBC (many regimens will work in 7 days), the addition of two antibacterials such as amoxycillin or clarithromycin and metronidazole or tinidazole. No other triple therapy regimens have currently been widely validated. If patients cannot tolerate any of these combinations because of side-effects or because of antibiotic allergy, bismuth triple therapy is a possible alternative; perhaps bismuth, tetracycline or amoxycillin, and metronidazole, although few routinely use this currently.

Monitoring the results

Because of the variability in results achieved, it is important to check whether *H. pylori* has been successfully eradicated if methods exist locally to do so. Most find the ^{13}C urea breath test best for this purpose.

4.1.2 Suggested H. pylori eradication treatment for patients with duodenal ulcer disease

Firm recommendations from around the world

Confirm that diagnosis of ulcer has been made at some time (there is usually no necessity to confirm *H. pylori* status since almost all adults with DU and the majority of those with GU are positive).

Report of the American Digestive Health Foundation

USA

FDA-approved treatment regimens for *H. pylori* infection are as follows.

• Omeprazole 40 mg od + clarithromycin 500 mg tid for 2 weeks, then omeprazole 20 mg od for 2 weeks.
• RBC 400 mg bid + clarithromycin 500 mg tid for 2 weeks, then RBC 400 mg bid for 2 weeks.
• Pepto-Bismol 525 mg qid + metronidazole 250 mg qid + tetracycline 500 mg qid for 2 weeks + H$_2$RA therapy as directed for 4 weeks.

- Lansoprazole 30 mg + amoxicillin 1 g + clarithromycin 500 mg bid for 2 weeks.

The following are promising therapies under evaluation.
- Omeprazole 20 mg + amoxicillin 1 g + clarithromycin 500 mg bid × 2 weeks.
- Omeprazole 20 mg or lansoprazole 30 mg + metronidazole 500 mg + clarithromycin 500 mg bid for 2 weeks.
- RBC 400 mg + amoxicillin 1 g + clarithromycin 500 mg bid for 2 weeks.
- RBC 400 mg metronidazole 500 mg + clarithromycin 500 mg bid for 2 weeks.

Report of the Asia Pacific Consensus Conference

Treatment regimens that attain eradication rates of 90% or greater by per-protocol analysis and 80% or greater by intent-to-treat analysis are recommended for *H. pylori* infection.

Asia Pacific
- PPI in standard dose bid + clarithromycin 500 mg bid + amoxicillin 1000 mg bid.
- PPI in standard dose bid + clarithromycin 500 mg bid + metronidazole 400 mg bid.
- RBC 400 mg bid + clarithromycin 500 mg bid + amoxicillin 1000 mg bid.
- RBC 400 mg bid + clarithromycin 500 mg bid + metronidazole 400 mg bid.

Each of the above regimens should be given for 7 days.

The Maastricht Consensus Report

European
One-week triple therapy using PPI bid *plus*:
- metronidazole 400 mg bid or tinidazole 500 mg bid plus clarithromycin 250 mg bid *or*;
- amoxycillin 1000 mg bid plus clarithromycin 500 mg bid *or*;
- amoxycillin 500 mg tid plus metronidazole 400 mg tid.

Classical bismuth-based triple therapy has been superseded by PPI-based triple therapy. Quadruple therapy, i.e. PPI + classical triple, can be used for triple therapy failure.

4.1.3 Recommended H. pylori eradication regimen

Opinions vary around the world and in this area are constantly changing. Nevertheless, at present a reasonable consensus for active or past documented peptic ulceration would be 1-week triple therapy consisting of:

- a PPI (omeprazole 40 mg/lansoprazole 30 mg or RBC 400 mg bid) *plus*;
- amoxycillin 1 g (some recommend bid) or clarithromycin 500 mg bid *plus*;
- metronidazole 400 mg bid or tinidazole 500 mg bid.

If patient remains *H. pylori* positive by carbon urea-labelled breath test *more than* 4 weeks after discontinuation of previous treatment course:

- quadruple therapy (PPI plus classical, i.e. bismuth-based triple therapy).

4.2 Patients with dyspepsia

The evidence for *H. pylori* playing a role in causing reflux oesophagitis or gastro-oesophageal reflux disease is at present non-existent and, in NUD, is confusing and uncertain. Few working in the field would currently advocate attempts at *H. pylori* eradication in these situations, or to ward off risk of subsequent gastric cancer development. Neither is the incidental discovery of *H. pylori* gastritis accepted as an indication for attempts at eradication therapy. The potential risks of treatment at present appear to outweigh any likely short- or long-term benefits in these groups (see Table 22).

In gastro-oesophageal reflux disease (GORD), the symptomatic benefits of antacid/alginate combinations, together with lifestyle advice, including losing weight, stopping smoking and maintenance of posture, are well established. Similarly, the proven healing benefits of acid suppressants, especially the PPIs omeprazole, lansoprazole and pantoprazole in severe disease, and the H_2RAs in milder disease, are generally accepted. Additional benefits can also be anticipated with prokinetics such as cisapride. It is also apparent that laparoscopic surgery (principally fundoplication) available in some centres, is encouraging a resurgence of interest in operative management, especially for those younger patients otherwise likely to continue on life-long acid suppressants (Table 23).

Long-term acid suppression in those with reflux who are *H. pylori* positive

There is concern that patients on long-term PPI treatment for GORD who are *H. pylori* positive may be at risk of developing gastric atrophy. There is no general agreement on these risks or whether *H. pylori* eradication should be achieved before starting long-term medical treatment. At

Table 23 Suggested management of oesophageal reflux disease.

Patient	Action
Symptomatic	Treat • antacid/alginate combination • if ineffective, H₂RA • healing course 6–8 weeks Supportive advice • lose weight • stop smoking • avoid bending • sleep upright • avoid tight clothes • small frequent meals • avoid late night eating • reduce chocolate, fat, alcohol, etc.
Endoscopic severe oesophagitis with persistent symptoms	Treat • PPI/H₂RA (×4 daily dosage is required in some patients with H₂RAs) • Healing course 4–6 weeks
Persistent symptoms/vomiting	Consider adding prokinetic agent, i.e. cisapride, domperidone, metoclopramide, etc. Exclude stricture/neoplasm
Maintenance required	Treat • Antacid/alginates, prokinetic agents Consider • H₂RAs long term/PPI • testing for *H. pylori* and eradicating infection if present (see text for explanation)
Intractable symptoms	Confirm diagnosis endoscopically Consider referral to gastroenterologist
An alternative to long-term maintenance treatment or for continuing unrelieved symptoms	Consider laparoscopic fundoplication

present it appears prudent to attempt this but it is not known whether this is beneficial.

For patients with NUD, antacids and H_2RAs cimetidine or ranitidine may be worthwhile, or consideration given to using a prokinetic such as cisapride or domperidone. Lifestyle advice may also be helpful for the long term, since relapse is not infrequent (Table 24).

4.3 Where are we going in the future?

Few can doubt the importance of the discovery of *H. pylori* (Fig. 22). It will probably be seen as one of the ironies of history that this bacterium was overlooked for so long and interest so focused elsewhere in our search for a cause for peptic ulceration. Nevertheless, there is often a temptation, when confronted by the realization of some of our oversights, to overreact and, in the case of *H. pylori*, it is tempting to attribute to it a role as a causative factor in a range of previously ill-understood disorders. At present the 'jury remains out' with most of these suggestions, the clear exceptions being active chronic gastritis, peptic ulcer disease and probably mucosa-associated lymphoid tissue (MALT) lymphoma. There is now overwhelming evidence that this organism plays a role in the initial development

Many unanswered
questions

Table 24 Non-ulcer dyspepsia.

Patient	Action
Symptomatic patient often with endoscopic evidence of gastritis or duodenitis	Treat • antacid: if ineffective, add H_2RA 4–6 weeks Supportive advice • stop smoking • reduce alcohol ingestion • avoid aggravating foods, i.e. fat, etc. • eat small, frequent meals
Persistent symptoms	Consider alternative treatment • sucralfate/bismuth • prokinetic agent, i.e. cisapride/domperidone • *H. pylori* eradication Consider alternative diagnoses: • gallstones, irritable bowel, etc. Consider referral to gastroenterologist

H. pylori is a common worldwide pathogen

- As such it appears to present a major public health risk, especially in some areas of the developing world

Fig. 22 *H. pylori* as a health problem.

and subsequent recurrence of these common and some less common diseases.

Nevertheless, from what we do know, the question of whether we should try and eradicate *H. pylori* should always be addressed in any patient with peptic ulceration and MALT lymphoma.

Treatment still needs improvement — but it is getting there!

Our greatest problem at present in the management of *H. pylori*-related disease is the limitations of much currently available treatment. Although very good results have been reported with a range of therapeutic combinations, none at present appears universally successful. We understand some of the reasons for this, but certainly not all and currently many would urge caution before adopting widespread attempts at eradication of this organism. The risks of side-effects (some serious), expense, inconvenience and possibilities of inducing bacterial resistance are amongst some of

We are still not ready to treat all infected individuals

the most cited and obvious reasons. Although progress is being made in achieving better responses to treatment, this is at the expense of adding more drugs to the treatment regimens. We appear some distance from achieving the ideal of a 'magic bullet' single drug for *H. pylori* eradication. One of the most encouraging aspects in this field is that we are starting to see the development of new drugs specifically targeted at *H. pylori* eradication. Only by moving forward in this way can we hope to fully understand the importance of this bacterium in human disease.

Perhaps we can immunize

For the future, the prospect of immunization against the organism seems an ideal worth striving for. To date, in a mouse model, the cat equivalent organism (*Helicobacter felis*) has been shown to induce protection when immunization is given with an added adjuvant. This provides hope that similar protection might develop in humans and, presumably if given early in childhood, may prevent subsequent infection, peptic ulceration and possibly gastric cancer. Unfortunately, even if the technical difficulties of

Who can afford it? immunization could be overcome, it is not entirely clear whether the economic problems of wide-scale immunization would be surmountable. Many of the epidemiological features of *H. pylori* infection mirror those of infectious hepatitis and immunization would need to be undertaken on a similar large scale. It is likely in both examples that those who most need it are the poorest and least able to afford it.

Much to discover Nevertheless, whatever the future brings for *H. pylori* research and especially in the treatment of this unusual organism, undoubtedly much excitement and intrigue lies ahead for all who have an interest in this topic.

Index